Blood Type RH Negative Diet Book

Becky Shelby

Table of Contents

Introduction..1

    Understanding the RH Negative Blood Type 3

    The Importance of Blood Type in Nutrition 5

    How the Blood Type Diet Works, Including RH
Negative 8

Chapter 1: RH Negative Blood Type Overview 11

    Characteristics and Traits of RH Negative Individuals
....14

    Health Considerations for RH Negative Blood Types
....17

Chapter 2: Blood Type Diet Fundamentals for RH
Negative Individuals 21

    Beneficial Foods for RH Negative Blood Types 21

    Foods to Avoid for RH Negative Individuals 24

Chapter 3: Sample Meal Plans for RH Negative Blood
Types...28

    Breakfast Options for RH Negative Blood Types.....28

    Lunch Options for RH Negative Blood Types..........39

Dinner Options for RH Negative Blood Types.........51

Snack and Dessert Options for RH Negative Blood Types...62

Seven day meal plan 71

Conclusion 74

About the author 76

My Little Request 78

Introduction

Dear Readers,

Welcome to the pages of "Blood Type RH Negative Diet Book." As you embark on this journey towards understanding the profound connection between your RH Negative blood type and the foods you consume, I extend my heartfelt gratitude for joining me on this exploration of health, wellness, and self-discovery.

The notion that our blood type can influence our well-being is a captivating concept that has gained recognition in recent years. For those with the RH Negative blood type, this book is designed to be a guiding light, offering insights into a personalized approach to nutrition that aligns with your unique biological makeup.

As we delve into the intricacies of the RH Negative blood type and its relationship with dietary choices, I invite you to approach this journey with an open heart and a willingness to embrace positive changes. This book is not just a collection of guidelines but a companion on your path to better health, providing practical advice, delicious recipes, and a sense of empowerment.

Throughout these pages, we will navigate the fundamentals of the Blood Type Diet, exploring the specific needs and considerations for individuals with RH Negative blood types. From beneficial foods to avoid, to sample meal plans tailored for your blood type, we will cover a spectrum of information aimed at helping you make informed and health-conscious decisions.

As you read the stories of others who have embraced the Blood Type Diet with RH Negative blood types, I hope you find inspiration and motivation to embark on your own transformative journey. Every person's experience is unique, and within these anecdotes lie the potential for newfound vitality and well-being.

This book is not just about what you eat; it's about cultivating a deeper connection with your body, understanding its signals, and making choices that resonate with your individuality. So, let's embark on this empowering expedition together, discovering the remarkable synergy between your RH Negative blood type and the nourishment that fuels your body and soul.

Wishing you health, happiness, and a fulfilling journey,

Becky Shelby

Author of "Blood Type RH Negative Diet Book "

Understanding the RH Negative Blood Type

The concept of blood types has fascinated scientists and health enthusiasts alike for decades. Among the various blood types, the RH factor adds an additional layer of complexity and intrigue to this biological puzzle. The RH factor refers to the presence or absence of a specific antigen, known as the Rhesus factor, on the surface of red blood cells. Individuals who have this antigen are classified as RH positive, while those lacking it are identified as RH negative.

For those who are RH negative, this blood type is somewhat enigmatic and represents a smaller percentage of the global population compared to RH positive individuals. The precise origins and evolutionary significance of RH negative blood types remain unclear, adding an element of mystery to this particular blood group.

Geneticists and anthropologists have explored various theories to explain the presence of RH negative blood types, ranging from ancient genetic mutations to extraterrestrial influences. While the scientific community continues to investigate these theories, the medical implications of RH negative blood types are a subject of growing interest.

Health considerations for RH negative individuals extend beyond blood transfusions and pregnancy complications. Some studies suggest potential associations between RH negative blood types and certain health conditions, such as autoimmune disorders, allergies, and sensitivities. However, it's crucial to approach these findings with caution, as more research is needed to establish conclusive links.

In the realm of nutrition, the Blood Type Diet has gained popularity as a personalized approach that considers an individual's blood type when recommending dietary choices. For RH negative individuals, understanding the nuances of this blood type can offer insights into optimal nutrition tailored to their specific needs.

Exploring the RH negative blood type involves delving into the unique characteristics and traits associated with these individuals. From physical attributes to potential health considerations, the RH negative blood type adds a layer of complexity to the understanding of human genetics and biology.

As we journey through this exploration, it's essential to approach the topic with a balanced perspective, appreciating the intricacies of human diversity and the ongoing scientific inquiry that seeks to unravel the mysteries surrounding RH negative blood types. Whether you are an individual with an RH negative blood type or someone curious about the diversity within our species, understanding the RH negative blood type contributes to a richer tapestry of human biology and health.

The Importance of Blood Type in Nutrition

The notion that blood type could influence dietary needs and health outcomes is a captivating concept that has gained attention in recent years. The idea is central to the Blood Type Diet, a nutritional approach that posits that an individual's blood type should play a significant role in determining their optimal diet. While the scientific community may not universally endorse the Blood Type Diet, exploring the potential connections between blood type and nutrition can be enlightening.

1. Biochemical Individuality:

   - Each person is biochemically unique, and factors such as genetics, environment, and lifestyle contribute to this individuality. Blood type is one aspect of this biochemical makeup that proponents of the Blood Type Diet argue should be considered when crafting dietary recommendations.

2. Blood Type Antigens:

 - Blood types are determined by the presence or absence of specific antigens on the surface of red blood cells. The Blood Type Diet suggests that these antigens can react differently to certain foods, influencing digestion, nutrient absorption, and overall well-being.

3. Digestive Enzymes and Blood Type:

 - The Blood Type Diet proposes that individuals with different blood types may produce varying amounts of digestive enzymes. For example, individuals with blood type O are said to produce higher levels of stomach acid, making them better suited for a diet rich in proteins but limited in grains.

4. Inflammatory Response:

 - Proponents of the Blood Type Diet argue that certain foods may trigger an inflammatory response in individuals based on their blood type. By avoiding these triggering foods, individuals may experience improved digestion, reduced inflammation, and enhanced overall health.

5. Energy Levels and Blood Type:

 - The Blood Type Diet suggests that different blood types may have different energy requirements. For instance, individuals with blood type A are recommended a plant-based diet, while those with blood type O are advised to include more animal proteins. These recommendations aim to align with the energy needs of each blood type.

6. Potential Allergies and Sensitivities:

   - Some proponents of the Blood Type Diet argue that individuals with certain blood types may be more prone to allergies and sensitivities to specific foods. Tailoring the diet to the individual's blood type is believed to mitigate these potential issues.

It's important to note that the scientific community has not universally accepted the Blood Type Diet, and research supporting its claims is limited. As with any dietary approach, individual responses can vary, and the overall quality of one's diet, including factors like balance, variety, and moderation, remains crucial.

While the scientific validity of the Blood Type Diet is still a topic of debate, exploring the potential connections between blood type and nutrition can be a fascinating journey, offering insights into the intricate relationship between our biological makeup and the foods we consume.

How the Blood Type Diet Works, Including RH Negative

The Blood Type Diet, developed by Dr. Peter D'Adamo, proposes that an individual's blood type influences how their body reacts to certain foods and, subsequently, their overall health. The theory suggests that by aligning dietary choices with one's blood type, individuals can optimize digestion, enhance nutrient absorption, and reduce the risk of various health issues. When it comes to the RH negative blood type, the principles of the Blood Type Diet are applied similarly, with additional considerations for the unique characteristics of RH negative individuals.

1. Identification of Blood Type:

   - The first step in the Blood Type Diet is to determine one's blood type (A, B, AB, or O) and Rh factor (positive or negative). This information forms the basis for personalized dietary recommendations.

2. Food Lists for Each Blood Type:

   - The diet provides specific food lists for each blood type, categorizing foods as highly beneficial, neutral, or to be avoided. For RH negative individuals, these lists are tailored to account for the unique characteristics associated with this blood type.

3. Highly Beneficial Foods:

   - RH negative individuals are recommended to emphasize foods classified as highly beneficial for their blood type. These are foods believed to enhance overall well-being and support the specific needs associated with RH negative blood types. For instance, RH negative individuals might be advised to include certain types of meat, fish, fruits, and vegetables in their diet.

4. Neutral Foods:

   - Neutral foods are considered generally safe for consumption and are not expected to have a significant impact on health for individuals with a specific blood type. RH negative individuals may find a variety of options in this category that can be included in their meals without major concerns.

5. Foods to Avoid:

   - The diet also identifies foods that individuals should avoid, as they are believed to be less compatible with the digestive and metabolic characteristics associated with specific blood types. RH negative individuals may be cautioned against certain foods that could potentially have adverse effects on their health.

6. Exercise Recommendations:

   - In addition to dietary guidelines, the Blood Type Diet incorporates exercise recommendations tailored to each blood type. Regular physical activity is considered essential for overall health, and RH negative individuals may benefit from exercises that align with their blood type.

7. Mind-Body Connection:

   - The Blood Type Diet extends beyond food and exercise, emphasizing the mind-body connection. Stress management techniques and lifestyle recommendations are included, recognizing that factors beyond diet can impact health and well-being.

It's important to note that while some individuals report positive experiences with the Blood Type Diet, scientific support for its principles is limited. RH negative individuals, like those with other blood types, are encouraged to approach this dietary approach with an open mind and consult with healthcare professionals to ensure that their nutritional needs are met in a balanced and evidence-based manner.

Chapter 1: RH Negative Blood Type Overview

The RH negative blood type, also known as Rhesus negative, refers to individuals whose red blood cells lack the Rhesus factor (Rh factor or D antigen) on their surface. This factor is a protein that can be present or absent in people's blood, leading to the classification of two main blood types: RH positive and RH negative.

Comprehensive overview of the RH negative blood type:

1. Prevalence:

  - RH negative blood type is less common globally compared to RH positive. The percentage of people with RH negative blood types varies by population and ethnicity, with higher prevalence among certain groups.

2. Genetic Inheritance:

  - The RH factor is inherited from both parents. If both parents are RH negative, their offspring will also be RH negative. If at least one parent is RH positive, there is a possibility of having an RH positive child.

3. Blood Typing System:

  - The ABO blood group system classifies blood into four main types: A, B, AB, and O. The RH factor is an additional component, leading to eight possible blood types: A+, A-, B+, B-, AB+, AB-, O+, and O-. RH negative individuals can have any of the ABO blood types without the Rh factor.

4. Physiological Characteristics:

   - Individuals with RH negative blood type may share certain physiological characteristics. While these characteristics are not universal, some studies suggest potential associations between RH negative blood types and specific traits, such as heightened sensitivity to environmental factors.

5. Pregnancy Considerations:

   - RH negative individuals may face unique considerations during pregnancy. If an RH negative woman is carrying an RH positive baby, there is a risk of Rh incompatibility, which can lead to hemolytic disease of the newborn (HDN). To prevent complications, Rh-negative pregnant women may receive Rh immunoglobulin (RhIg) injections.

6. Health Associations:

   - Some studies have explored potential associations between RH negative blood types and certain health conditions. These include autoimmune disorders, allergies, and sensitivities. However, it's crucial to approach these findings with caution, as more research is needed to establish conclusive links.

7. Blood Transfusions:

   - RH negative individuals can receive blood from both RH negative and RH positive donors. However, they are often considered universal plasma donors, meaning their plasma can be used for individuals of any blood type.

8. Evolutionary Theories:

   - The origins of the RH negative blood type remain a subject of interest and speculation. Some theories propose ancient genetic mutations, while others delve into more unconventional hypotheses, including extraterrestrial influences. These theories are not widely accepted within the scientific community.

Understanding the RH negative blood type involves considering both the biological aspects and potential health implications associated with this less common blood group. While the scientific community continues to explore the intricacies of blood types, RH negative individuals can rely on medical guidance and healthcare professionals for personalized health recommendations.

Characteristics and Traits of RH Negative Individuals

The characteristics and traits associated with RH negative individuals have been a subject of interest and speculation. While it's important to note that these traits are not universally applicable, some studies and anecdotal evidence suggest certain commonalities. It's crucial to approach these observations with caution, as individual variations within any blood type are significant, and scientific consensus on these traits is still evolving. Here are some characteristics and traits that have been associated with RH negative individuals:

1. Sensitivity to Environmental Factors:

   - Some studies and anecdotal reports propose that RH negative individuals may exhibit heightened sensitivity to environmental factors, such as temperature, light, and sound. They may perceive and react to these stimuli more intensely than individuals with RH positive blood types.

2. Intuition and Empathy:

   - Some proponents suggest that RH negative individuals may possess a heightened sense of intuition and empathy. They may be more attuned to emotional cues and exhibit a strong sense of compassion.

3. Spiritual and Creative Inclinations:

   - There are claims that RH negative individuals may have a proclivity towards spirituality and creativity. Some believe that they are more likely to be drawn to artistic pursuits and have a deep connection to spiritual or metaphysical concepts.

4. Low Blood Pressure:

   - Some studies have suggested a potential association between RH negative blood types and lower blood pressure. However, individual health factors, lifestyle, and genetics can also play significant roles in blood pressure levels.

5. Prevalence in Certain Ethnic Groups:

   - RH negative blood types are found in varying frequencies among different ethnic groups. Some studies have shown higher prevalence in populations with European ancestry, but the distribution can differ globally.

6. Adaptability to Different Environments:

   - Anecdotal accounts suggest that RH negative individuals may demonstrate adaptability to diverse environments. Some proponents propose that this adaptability could be linked to ancient migrations and evolutionary factors.

7. Tendency Toward Psychic Phenomena:

   - In some alternative and metaphysical circles, RH negative individuals are associated with a higher likelihood of experiencing psychic phenomena or having paranormal experiences. However, these claims lack empirical scientific support.

8. Challenges in Pregnancy:

   - RH negative women may face challenges during pregnancy, particularly if carrying an RH positive baby. Rh incompatibility can lead to complications, and Rh-negative pregnant women may receive Rh immunoglobulin (RhIg) injections to prevent issues.

It's important to approach these characteristics with critical thinking and an understanding that individual experiences and traits can vary widely. While the scientific community acknowledges the unique aspects of RH negative blood types, definitive evidence supporting these specific traits is still lacking. The study of blood types and their potential associations with various traits remains an area of ongoing research and exploration.

Health Considerations for RH Negative Blood Types

Health considerations for RH negative blood types involve examining potential associations between this blood type and certain health conditions. It's important to note that while some studies and theories propose links between RH negative blood types and specific health factors, the scientific evidence supporting these associations is limited and not universally accepted. Individuals with RH negative blood types should prioritize overall health and consult with healthcare professionals for personalized advice. Here are some health considerations associated with RH negative blood types:

1. Pregnancy Complications:

  - One of the most well-established health considerations for RH negative individuals is the risk of Rh incompatibility during pregnancy. If an RH negative woman is carrying an RH positive baby, there is a potential risk of hemolytic disease of the newborn (HDN). To prevent complications, Rh-negative pregnant women are often administered Rh immunoglobulin (RhIg) injections.

2. Autoimmune Disorders:

   - Some studies and anecdotal reports suggest potential associations between RH negative blood types and autoimmune disorders. These conditions involve the immune system mistakenly attacking the body's own tissues. However, more research is needed to establish conclusive links.

3. Allergies and Sensitivities:

   - There are claims that RH negative individuals may be more prone to allergies and sensitivities. This speculation is based on the idea that the immune system in RH negative individuals might react differently to certain environmental factors. Scientific evidence supporting this notion is limited.

4. Lower Incidence of Cardiovascular Diseases:

   - Some studies have suggested a lower incidence of cardiovascular diseases in individuals with RH negative blood types. However, the relationship between blood type and cardiovascular health is complex and influenced by various factors, including lifestyle and genetics.

5. Heightened Sensitivity to Environmental Factors:

   - RH negative individuals are sometimes associated with heightened sensitivity to environmental factors, such as changes in temperature, light, and sound.

However, scientific evidence supporting these claims is limited, and individual variations play a significant role.

6. Possible Associations with Certain Cancers:

  - Limited studies have explored potential associations between RH negative blood types and specific types of cancer. However, these findings are preliminary, and more research is needed to establish conclusive links between blood type and cancer susceptibility.

7. Adaptability to Different Environments:

  - Some anecdotal accounts suggest that RH negative individuals may exhibit adaptability to diverse environments. This adaptability is theorized to be linked to ancient migrations and evolutionary factors, but scientific support for this idea is speculative.

8. Potential Impact on Immune Response:

  - The immune system's response to infections and diseases may vary among individuals with different blood types. Some studies propose that the immune response in RH negative individuals could differ, but more research is required to substantiate these claims.

It's crucial for individuals with RH negative blood types to prioritize general health practices, including a balanced diet, regular exercise, and routine healthcare check-ups. While intriguing, the associations mentioned above should be approached with caution until further research establishes more concrete links between RH negative blood types and specific health considerations. Always consult with healthcare professionals for personalized health advice.

Chapter 2: Blood Type Diet Fundamentals for RH Negative Individuals

Beneficial Foods for RH Negative Blood Types

The Blood Type Diet suggests that individuals with different blood types should consume specific foods that are considered beneficial for their blood type. While scientific support for the Blood Type Diet is limited, and individual responses to foods can vary, here are general recommendations for beneficial foods for RH negative blood types:

1. Lean Protein:

  - RH negative individuals, particularly those with blood type O, are often advised to include lean protein sources in their diet. This may include poultry, fish, and lean cuts of pork. These protein sources are believed to be well-tolerated by individuals with RH negative blood types.

2. Seafood:

  - Fish, especially cold-water varieties rich in omega-3 fatty acids, is often recommended for RH negative individuals. Salmon, mackerel, and trout are examples of fish that may be considered beneficial.

3. Leafy Green Vegetables:

  - Dark, leafy green vegetables are generally encouraged for individuals with RH negative blood types. This includes spinach, kale, and Swiss chard, which are rich in vitamins, minerals, and antioxidants.

4. Berries:

  - Berries, such as blueberries, strawberries, and raspberries, are often suggested for RH negative individuals. These fruits are considered rich in antioxidants and may provide health benefits.

5. Pineapple:

  - Some proponents of the Blood Type Diet recommend pineapple for RH negative individuals. It is believed to be beneficial for certain blood types and may contribute to digestive health.

6. Olive Oil:

  - Olive oil is often promoted as a healthy fat source for individuals with RH negative blood types. It is considered a monounsaturated fat that may have cardiovascular benefits.

7. Garlic and Onions:

  - Garlic and onions are commonly included in the diet recommendations for RH negative individuals. They are believed to offer immune-boosting properties and may be flavorful additions to meals.

8. Moderate Dairy:

  - Depending on the specific blood type, moderate consumption of dairy products such as yogurt, kefir, and certain cheeses may be recommended. RH negative individuals are typically advised to choose dairy options that align with their blood type.

9. Green Tea:

  - Green tea is often suggested for its potential health benefits, including antioxidants. It is considered a suitable beverage choice for individuals with RH negative blood types.

10. Turkey:

  - Turkey is commonly recommended as a protein source for certain blood types within the RH negative group. It is considered a lean meat option.

It's important to note that these recommendations are based on the principles of the Blood Type Diet and may not be supported by robust scientific evidence. Additionally, individual responses to foods can vary, and dietary needs are influenced by various factors beyond blood type. It is advisable for individuals to consult with healthcare professionals or registered dietitians for personalized nutrition guidance based on their specific health status, preferences, and lifestyle.

Foods to Avoid for RH Negative Individuals

The Blood Type Diet proposes that individuals with different blood types should avoid certain foods that may not be well-tolerated or may have adverse effects on their health. While the scientific support for the Blood Type Diet is limited, and individual responses to foods can vary, here are general recommendations for foods to avoid for RH negative blood types:

1. Red Meat:

   - Some versions of the Blood Type Diet suggest that individuals with RH negative blood types, particularly blood type A, should limit or avoid red meat. This includes beef and lamb, as these meats are believed to be less compatible with certain blood types.

2. Processed Meats:

   - Processed meats, such as sausages, hot dogs, and bacon, are often advised against for individuals with RH negative blood types. They may contain additives and preservatives that are considered less suitable for certain blood types.

3. High-Fat Dairy:

   - Certain blood types within the RH negative group are recommended to limit high-fat dairy products, such as whole milk, full-fat yogurt, and certain cheeses. Instead, they may opt for moderate or low-fat dairy options.

4. Wheat and Gluten-Containing Grains:

   - Individuals with RH negative blood types, particularly blood type O, may be advised to limit or avoid wheat and gluten-containing grains. This includes foods like wheat bread, pasta, and cereals.

5. Corn and Corn Products:

   - Corn and corn-based products may be discouraged for some RH negative blood types. This includes cornmeal, corn syrup, and certain snacks made from corn.

6. Certain Beans and Legumes:

   - Some versions of the Blood Type Diet recommend avoiding certain beans and legumes for individuals with RH negative blood types. This may include kidney beans, lentils, and peanuts.

7. Certain Fruits:

   - Depending on the specific blood type, there may be recommendations to limit or avoid certain fruits. For example, individuals with RH negative blood types may be advised to avoid oranges or tomatoes.

8. Unhealthy Fats:

Examples: Trans fats and excessive saturated fats. Sources of unhealthy fats include fried foods, processed snacks, and some baked goods. It's generally recommended to limit these fats for heart health.

9. Shellfish:

   - Shellfish, including oysters, crabs, and clams, may be advised against for certain blood types within the RH negative group. These foods are considered less compatible for some individuals.

10. Certain Nuts and Seeds:

   - Some versions of the Blood Type Diet recommend avoiding specific nuts and seeds. For example, individuals with RH negative blood types may be advised to limit cashews or peanuts.

It's important to approach these recommendations with caution, as the scientific evidence supporting the Blood Type Diet is limited, and individual responses to foods can vary widely. Additionally, individuals with RH negative blood types should prioritize a well-balanced diet that meets their nutritional needs. Consulting with healthcare professionals or registered dietitians is recommended for personalized nutrition guidance based on individual health status, preferences, and lifestyle.

Chapter 3: Sample Meal Plans for RH Negative Blood Types

While the Blood Type Diet recommends specific foods for different blood types, it's important to note that scientific evidence supporting these recommendations is limited. Additionally, individual responses to foods can vary. Below are food options that align with the general principles of the Blood Type Diet, with the most suitable negative blood type for each.

Breakfast Options for RH Negative Blood Types

1. Omelette with Spinach and Turkey (Blood Type O):

   - A protein-packed breakfast option for individuals with blood type O. Include spinach for added nutrients and flavor.

   Ingredients:

   - 2 large eggs

   - 1 cup fresh spinach, chopped

   - 50g turkey breast, cooked and diced

   - Salt and pepper to taste

- Olive oil for cooking

Instructions:

1. In a bowl, whisk the eggs and season with salt and pepper.

2. Heat olive oil in a non-stick skillet over medium heat.

3. Add chopped spinach to the skillet and sauté until wilted.

4. Pour the whisked eggs over the spinach.

5. Sprinkle diced turkey evenly over the eggs.

6. Cook until the edges start to set, then gently lift the edges and tilt the pan to let uncooked eggs flow underneath.

7. Once the omelette is set, fold it in half and serve hot.

2. Greek Yogurt Parfait with Berries (Blood Type A):

- A breakfast option rich in probiotics from Greek yogurt, suitable for individuals with blood type A. Add berries for antioxidants and natural sweetness.

Ingredients:

- 1 cup Greek yogurt

- 1/2 cup mixed berries (blueberries, strawberries, raspberries)

- 1 tablespoon honey

- 2 tablespoons granola

Instructions:

1. In a glass or bowl, layer Greek yogurt at the bottom.

2. Add a layer of mixed berries on top of the yogurt.

3. Drizzle honey over the berries.

4. Sprinkle granola on the honey layer.

5. Repeat the layers if desired.

6. Serve immediately and enjoy the parfait.

3. Smoked Salmon and Avocado Toast (Blood Type B):

- A nutrient-dense breakfast with omega-3 fatty acids from salmon, suitable for individuals with blood type B. Avocado provides healthy fats.

Ingredients:

- 2 slices whole-grain bread

- 1/2 avocado, mashed

- 50g smoked salmon

- Fresh dill for garnish

- Lemon wedges (optional)

Instructions:

1. Toast the slices of whole-grain bread.

2. Spread mashed avocado evenly over each slice.

3. Arrange smoked salmon on top of the avocado.

4. Garnish with fresh dill.

5. Squeeze lemon juice over the top if desired.

6. Serve the smoked salmon and avocado toast immediately.

4. Quinoa Breakfast Bowl with Fruit (Blood Type AB):

- A balanced breakfast with quinoa, a complete protein, suitable for individuals with blood type AB. Top with a variety of fruits for vitamins and minerals.

Ingredients:

- 1/2 cup cooked quinoa

- 1/4 cup sliced strawberries

- 1/4 cup blueberries

- 1 tablespoon chopped nuts (almonds, walnuts)

- 1 tablespoon honey

- Greek yogurt (optional)

Instructions:

1. In a bowl, combine cooked quinoa, sliced strawberries, blueberries, and chopped nuts.

2. Drizzle honey over the top.

3. Optionally, add a dollop of Greek yogurt.

4. Stir gently to combine all ingredients.

5. Enjoy the quinoa breakfast bowl.

5. Almond Butter Banana Smoothie (Blood Type O):

- A protein-rich smoothie with almond butter, suitable for individuals with blood type O. Bananas add natural sweetness and potassium.

Ingredients:

- 1 banana, frozen

- 1 tablespoon almond butter

- 1 cup almond milk

- 1/2 teaspoon honey (optional)

- Ice cubes (optional)

Instructions:

1. Place the frozen banana, almond butter, and almond milk in a blender.

2. Add honey if additional sweetness is desired.

3. Blend until smooth and creamy.

4. If a colder consistency is preferred, add ice cubes and blend again.

5. Pour into a glass and enjoy the almond butter banana smoothie.

6. Chia Seed Pudding with Coconut Milk (Blood Type A):

- A plant-based and gluten-free option suitable for individuals with blood type A. Chia seeds provide omega-3 fatty acids and fiber.

Ingredients:

- 2 tablespoons chia seeds

- 1/2 cup coconut milk

- 1/2 teaspoon vanilla extract

- Fresh berries for topping

Instructions:

1. In a bowl, mix chia seeds, coconut milk, and vanilla extract.

2. Stir well to combine and ensure no clumps.

3. Refrigerate for at least 4 hours or overnight to allow the chia seeds to absorb the liquid and create a pudding-like consistency.

4. Before serving, top with fresh berries.

5. Stir gently and enjoy the chia seed pudding.

7. Egg White Veggie Scramble (Blood Type B):

- A low-fat breakfast option with egg whites and a variety of vegetables, suitable for individuals with blood type B.

Ingredients:

- 1 cup egg whites

- 1/2 cup bell peppers, diced

- 1/2 cup spinach, chopped

- 1/4 cup feta cheese, crumbled

- Salt and pepper to taste

- Olive oil for cooking

Instructions:

1. Heat olive oil in a skillet over medium heat.

2. Add diced bell peppers to the skillet and sauté until softened.

3. Add chopped spinach and cook until wilted.

4. Pour egg whites over the vegetables.

5. Stir gently until the eggs are cooked through.

6. Sprinkle crumbled feta cheese on top.

7. Season with salt and pepper to taste.

8. Serve the egg white veggie scramble hot.

8. Buckwheat Pancakes with Blueberries (Blood Type AB):

- Buckwheat is a non-wheat grain suitable for individuals with blood type AB. Top pancakes with blueberries for added antioxidants.

Ingredients:

- 1/2 cup buckwheat flour

- 1/2 teaspoon baking powder

- 1/4 teaspoon salt

- 1/2 cup almond milk

- 1 egg

- 1 tablespoon maple syrup

- 1/2 cup fresh blueberries

Instructions:

1. In a bowl, whisk together buckwheat flour, baking powder, and salt.

2. Add almond milk, egg, and maple syrup to the dry ingredients. Mix until well combined.

3. Fold in fresh blueberries.

4. Heat a griddle or non-stick pan over medium heat.

5. Pour 1/4 cup of batter onto the griddle for each pancake.

6. Cook until bubbles form on the surface, then flip and cook the other side.

7. Serve the buckwheat pancakes with additional blueberries.

9. Coconut Yogurt with Granola and Mango (Blood Type O):

- A dairy-free option with coconut yogurt, suitable for individuals with blood type O. Granola and mango add crunch and natural sweetness.

Ingredients:

- 1 cup coconut yogurt

- 1/2 cup granola

- 1/2 mango, diced

- 1 tablespoon shredded coconut

Instructions:

1. In a bowl, spoon coconut yogurt.

2. Top with granola, diced mango, and shredded coconut.

3. Mix gently to combine flavors.

4. Serve the coconut yogurt with granola and mango.

10. Turkey and Vegetable Breakfast Wrap (Blood Type B):

- A savory breakfast option with turkey and a variety of vegetables, suitable for individuals with blood type B. Use a lettuce wrap for a gluten-free option.

Ingredients:

- 1 whole-grain wrap or tortilla

- 2 large eggs, scrambled

- 50g turkey breast, cooked and sliced

- 1/4 cup bell peppers, diced

- 1/4 cup tomatoes, diced

- Fresh cilantro for garnish

- Salt and pepper to taste

Instructions:

1. In a skillet, scramble eggs until cooked through.

2. In the same skillet, briefly warm the whole-grain wrap.

3. Lay the warm wrap on a plate and add scrambled eggs in the center.

4. Top with sliced turkey, diced bell peppers, and tomatoes.

5. Season with salt and pepper to taste.

6. Garnish with fresh cilantro.

7. Fold the sides of the wrap, creating a breakfast burrito.

8. Serve the turkey and vegetable breakfast wrap warm.

These breakfast options aim to incorporate the general principles of the Blood Type Diet, but individual preferences and dietary tolerances should be considered. It's essential to prioritize a well-balanced diet that meets overall nutritional needs.

Lunch Options for RH Negative Blood Types

1. Grilled Chicken Salad with Mixed Greens (Blood Type O):

  - Grilled chicken breast served on a bed of mixed greens, including spinach and arugula. Add cherry tomatoes, cucumber, and a vinaigrette made with olive oil for a nutritious and satisfying lunch.

Ingredients:

- 1 boneless, skinless chicken breast

- Mixed greens (spinach, arugula, etc.)

- Cherry tomatoes, halved

- Cucumber, sliced

- Olive oil

- Balsamic vinegar

- Salt and pepper to taste

Instructions:

1. Season the chicken breast with salt and pepper.

2. Grill the chicken until fully cooked.

3. In a large bowl, combine mixed greens, cherry tomatoes, and cucumber.

4. Slice the grilled chicken and place it on top of the salad.

5. Drizzle with olive oil and balsamic vinegar.

6. Toss gently and enjoy the grilled chicken salad.

2. Vegetarian Quinoa Bowl (Blood Type A):

   - Quinoa mixed with sautéed vegetables such as bell
peppers, zucchini, and cherry tomatoes. Top with
avocado slices and a drizzle of lemon-tahini dressing for
a plant-based and protein-rich option.

   Ingredients:

   - 1 cup cooked quinoa

   - Mixed vegetables (bell peppers, zucchini, cherry
tomatoes)

   - Avocado, sliced

   - Lemon-tahini dressing (mix tahini, lemon juice, olive
oil)

   - Salt and pepper to taste

   Instructions:

   1. Sauté mixed vegetables until tender.

   2. In a bowl, combine cooked quinoa, sautéed
vegetables, and avocado slices.

   3. Drizzle with lemon-tahini dressing.

   4. Season with salt and pepper to taste.

   5. Toss gently and serve the vegetarian quinoa bowl.

3. Salmon Sushi Bowl (Blood Type B):

   - Cooked salmon chunks served over a bowl of sushi rice or cauliflower rice. Add seaweed, cucumber, and avocado slices. Drizzle with soy sauce or a tamari-based dressing for flavor.

   Ingredients:

   - Cooked salmon fillet, flaked

   - Sushi rice or cauliflower rice

   - Seaweed sheets, torn into pieces

   - Cucumber, sliced

   - Avocado, sliced

   - Soy sauce or tamari

   Instructions:

   1. Place sushi rice or cauliflower rice in a bowl.

   2. Arrange flaked salmon, torn seaweed, cucumber, and avocado on top.

   3. Drizzle with soy sauce or tamari.

   4. Gently mix and enjoy the salmon sushi bowl.

4. Chickpea and Vegetable Stir-Fry (Blood Type AB):

   - Stir-fried chickpeas with a colorful mix of vegetables like broccoli, bell peppers, and snap peas. Season with ginger, garlic, and a light soy sauce. Serve over brown rice or quinoa.

Ingredients:

  - 1 can chickpeas, drained and rinsed

  - Broccoli florets

  - Bell peppers, sliced

  - Soy sauce

  - Ginger, minced

  - Garlic, minced

  - Cooked brown rice or quinoa

Instructions:

  1. In a wok or skillet, stir-fry chickpeas, broccoli, and bell peppers.

  2. Add minced ginger and garlic.

  3. Drizzle with soy sauce.

  4. Stir until vegetables are tender.

  5. Serve over cooked brown rice or quinoa.

5. Turkey and Avocado Wrap (Blood Type O):

- Sliced turkey breast wrapped in a whole-grain tortilla with avocado, lettuce, and tomato. Add a spread of hummus for extra flavor and a boost of protein.

Ingredients:

- Sliced turkey breast

- Whole-grain tortilla

- Avocado, sliced

- Lettuce

- Tomato, sliced

- Hummus

Instructions:

1. Lay the whole-grain tortilla on a flat surface.

2. Spread a layer of hummus on the tortilla.

3. Add sliced turkey, avocado, lettuce, and tomato.

4. Roll the tortilla into a wrap.

5. Slice in half and enjoy the turkey and avocado wrap.

6. Mediterranean Lentil Salad (Blood Type A):

- Lentils tossed with cherry tomatoes, cucumbers, red onion, and Kalamata olives. Dress with olive oil, lemon juice, and a sprinkle of feta cheese for a Mediterranean-inspired lunch.

Ingredients:

- 1 cup cooked lentils

- Cherry tomatoes, halved

- Cucumber, diced

- Red onion, finely chopped

- Kalamata olives, sliced

- Feta cheese, crumbled

- Olive oil

- Lemon juice

- Salt and pepper to taste

Instructions:

1. In a bowl, combine cooked lentils, cherry tomatoes, cucumber, red onion, olives, and feta cheese.

2. Drizzle with olive oil and lemon juice.

3. Season with salt and pepper to taste.

4. Toss gently and serve the Mediterranean lentil salad.

7. Shrimp and Veggie Skewers (Blood Type B):

- Skewers with grilled shrimp, cherry tomatoes, and bell peppers. Serve with a side of quinoa or couscous and drizzle with a lemon-herb dressing.

Ingredients:

- Shrimp, peeled and deveined

- Cherry tomatoes

- Bell peppers, cut into chunks

- Olive oil

- Lemon juice

- Garlic, minced

- Fresh parsley, chopped

- Salt and pepper to taste

Instructions:

1. In a bowl, mix shrimp, cherry tomatoes, and bell peppers.

2. In a separate bowl, whisk together olive oil, lemon juice, minced garlic, chopped parsley, salt, and pepper.

3. Thread shrimp and vegetables onto skewers.

4. Grill or broil until shrimp are cooked.

5. Drizzle with the prepared dressing and serve the shrimp and veggie skewers.

8. Tofu and Broccoli Stir-Fry (Blood Type AB):

- Stir-fried tofu cubes with broccoli florets in a savory garlic and ginger sauce. Serve over brown rice or noodles for a satisfying and plant-based lunch option.

Ingredients:

- Firm tofu, cubed

- Broccoli florets

- Soy sauce

- Sesame oil

- Garlic, minced

- Ginger, minced

- Brown rice or noodles

Instructions:

1. In a wok or skillet, stir-fry tofu and broccoli.

2. In a small bowl, mix soy sauce, sesame oil, minced garlic, and minced ginger.

3. Add the sauce to the tofu and broccoli mixture.

4. Stir until everything is well-coated and heated through.

5. Serve over brown rice or noodles.

9. Chicken Caesar Salad with Kale (Blood Type O):

- Grilled chicken breast on a bed of kale, tossed with Caesar dressing, cherry tomatoes, and croutons. Opt for a dressing made with olive oil and lemon for a lighter version.

Ingredients:

- Grilled chicken breast, sliced

- Kale, chopped

- Croutons

- Parmesan cheese, shaved

- Caesar dressing (olive oil, lemon juice, Dijon mustard, garlic)

- Salt and pepper to taste

Instructions:

1. In a large bowl, combine chopped kale, grilled chicken, croutons, and shaved Parmesan cheese.

2. In a small bowl, whisk together ingredients for Caesar dressing.

3. Drizzle the dressing over the salad and toss to combine.

4. Season with salt and pepper to taste.

5. Enjoy the chicken Caesar salad with kale.

10. Eggplant and Chickpea Curry (Blood Type A):

- A flavorful curry made with eggplant, chickpeas, tomatoes, and a blend of spices. Serve over quinoa or basmati rice for a hearty and plant-based lunch.

Ingredients:

- Eggplant, cubed

- Chickpeas, cooked

- Tomatoes, diced

- Onion, finely chopped

- Curry powder

- Coconut milk

- Garlic, minced

- Ginger, minced

- Basmati rice

Instructions:

1. In a pot, sauté chopped onion, minced garlic, and minced ginger.

2. Add cubed eggplant, chickpeas, diced tomatoes, and curry powder.

3. Pour in coconut milk and let simmer until eggplant is tender.

4. Meanwhile, cook basmati rice according to package instructions.

5. Serve the eggplant and chickpea curry over the cooked basmati rice.

These lunch options aim to incorporate the general principles of the Blood Type Diet, but individual preferences and dietary tolerances should be considered. Adjustments can be made based on personal tastes and nutritional needs. Always consult with healthcare professionals or registered dietitians for personalized nutrition guidance.

Dinner Options for RH Negative Blood Types

1. Grilled Salmon with Asparagus (Blood Type O):

- Grilled salmon seasoned with herbs, served with roasted asparagus. This dinner is rich in omega-3 fatty acids and provides a balance of protein and vegetables.

Ingredients:

- Salmon fillets

- Fresh asparagus

- Olive oil

- Lemon juice

- Garlic powder

- Salt and pepper to taste

Instructions:

1. Preheat the grill.

2. Season salmon fillets with olive oil, lemon juice, garlic powder, salt, and pepper.

3. Grill salmon for 4-5 minutes per side or until cooked through.

4. Toss asparagus with olive oil, salt, and pepper.

5. Grill asparagus until tender-crisp.

6. Serve grilled salmon over a bed of grilled asparagus.

2. Vegetarian Stir-Fried Tofu and Broccoli (Blood Type A):

- Stir-fried tofu with broccoli, bell peppers, and snap peas in a light soy sauce. Served over brown rice or quinoa, this vegetarian option is packed with plant-based protein.

Ingredients:

- Firm tofu, cubed

- Broccoli florets

- Bell peppers, sliced

- Snap peas

- Soy sauce

- Ginger, minced

- Garlic, minced

- Brown rice or quinoa

Instructions:

1. In a wok or skillet, stir-fry tofu until golden.

2. Add broccoli, bell peppers, and snap peas. Continue stir-frying.

3. Mix in minced ginger and garlic.

4. Pour soy sauce over the mixture and stir until vegetables are tender.

5. Serve over brown rice or quinoa.

3. Turkey and Vegetable Skewers (Blood Type B):

- Skewers with marinated turkey breast, cherry tomatoes, and bell peppers. Grilled or baked, these skewers offer a mix of lean protein and colorful vegetables.

Ingredients:

- Turkey breast, cut into cubes

- Cherry tomatoes

- Bell peppers, cut into chunks

- Olive oil

- Lemon juice

- Oregano, dried or fresh

- Salt and pepper to taste

Instructions:

1. Preheat the grill or oven.

2. In a bowl, mix turkey cubes, cherry tomatoes, and bell peppers.

3. Drizzle with olive oil and lemon juice.

4. Season with oregano, salt, and pepper.

5. Thread the turkey and vegetables onto skewers.

6. Grill or bake until turkey is cooked through.

4. Quinoa Stuffed Bell Peppers (Blood Type AB):

- Bell peppers filled with a mixture of quinoa, black beans, tomatoes, and spices. Baked until tender, this dish provides a balanced blend of grains, protein, and veggies.

Ingredients:

- Bell peppers, halved and cleaned

- Quinoa, cooked

- Black beans, drained and rinsed

- Diced tomatoes

- Cumin, paprika, and chili powder to taste

- Shredded cheese (optional)

Instructions:

1. Preheat the oven.

2. In a bowl, mix cooked quinoa, black beans, diced tomatoes, and spices.

3. Stuff the bell peppers with the quinoa mixture.

4. Top with shredded cheese if desired.

5. Bake until peppers are tender.

5. Chicken and Vegetable Curry (Blood Type O):

- Chicken curry cooked with a variety of vegetables such as carrots, bell peppers, and spinach. Served with basmati rice or cauliflower rice for a flavorful and satisfying meal.

Ingredients:

- Chicken breasts, cubed

- Carrots, sliced

- Bell peppers, diced

- Spinach leaves

- Curry powder

- Coconut milk

- Basmati rice or cauliflower rice

Instructions:

1. In a pan, cook chicken until browned.

2. Add carrots, bell peppers, and spinach.

3. Sprinkle curry powder and stir.

4. Pour in coconut milk and let simmer until vegetables are tender.

5. Serve over basmati rice or cauliflower rice.

6. Mushroom and Spinach Frittata (Blood Type A):

- A frittata made with eggs, mushrooms, spinach, and herbs. Baked to perfection, this dish is a protein-rich and veggie-packed option.

Ingredients:

- Eggs

- Mushrooms, sliced

- Spinach, chopped

- Onion, diced

- Garlic, minced

- Olive oil

- Salt and pepper to taste

Instructions:

1. Preheat the oven.

2. In a skillet, sauté mushrooms, spinach, onion, and garlic in olive oil until softened.

3. In a bowl, whisk eggs and season with salt and pepper.

4. Pour the whisked eggs over the vegetables in the skillet.

5. Cook on the stovetop for a few minutes, then transfer to the oven to broil until the top is set.

7. Vegetarian Broccoli and Tofu Stir-Fry (Blood Type B):

- Stir-fried broccoli and tofu in a savory sauce with garlic and ginger. Served over brown rice or noodles, this vegetarian stir-fry is a delicious and nutritious choice.

Ingredients:

- Firm tofu, cubed

- Broccoli florets

- Soy sauce

- Sesame oil

- Ginger, minced

- Garlic, minced

- Brown rice or noodles

Instructions:

1. In a wok or skillet, stir-fry tofu and broccoli.

2. In a small bowl, mix soy sauce, sesame oil, minced ginger, and minced garlic.

3. Add the sauce to the tofu and broccoli mixture.

4. Stir until everything is well-coated and heated through.

5. Serve over brown rice or noodles.

8. Eggplant Parmesan (Blood Type AB):

- Baked eggplant slices layered with marinara sauce and mozzarella cheese. This vegetarian dish is served over whole-grain pasta for a comforting and satisfying dinner.

Ingredients:

- Eggplant, sliced

- Marinara sauce

- Mozzarella cheese, shredded

- Parmesan cheese, grated

- Italian seasoning

- Whole-grain pasta

Instructions:

1. Preheat the oven.

2. Layer sliced eggplant in a baking dish with marinara sauce, mozzarella, and Parmesan.

3. Repeat the layers, finishing with cheese on top.

4. Sprinkle with Italian seasoning.

5. Bake until bubbly and golden.

6. Serve over whole-grain pasta.

9. Lemon Herb Grilled Chicken with Quinoa (Blood Type O):

- Grilled chicken breasts marinated in lemon and herbs, served with fluffy quinoa. This dinner option is high in protein and provides a good source of complex carbohydrates.

Ingredients:

- Chicken breasts

- Lemon juice

- Fresh herbs (rosemary, thyme, oregano)

- Olive oil

- Garlic, minced

- Quinoa, cooked

Instructions:

1. In a bowl, mix lemon juice, fresh herbs, olive oil, and minced garlic.

2. Marinate chicken breasts in the mixture for at least 30 minutes.

3. Grill the chicken until fully cooked.

4. Serve the grilled chicken over a bed of cooked quinoa.

10. Shrimp and Avocado Salad (Blood Type B):

- Grilled shrimp served over a bed of mixed greens, avocado slices, and cherry tomatoes. Drizzled with a light vinaigrette, this salad offers a refreshing and protein-packed meal.

Ingredients:

- Shrimp, peeled and deveined

- Mixed greens

- Avocado, sliced

- Cherry tomatoes, halved

- Olive oil

- Lemon juice

- Dijon mustard

- Salt and pepper to taste

Instructions:

1. In a pan, cook shrimp until pink and opaque.

2. In a large bowl, toss mixed greens, avocado slices, and cherry tomatoes.

3. Whisk together olive oil, lemon juice, Dijon mustard, salt, and pepper for the dressing.

4. Top the salad with cooked shrimp and drizzle with the dressing.

Snack and Dessert Options for RH Negative Blood Types

Snack Options:

1. Greek Yogurt Parfait with Berries (Blood Type A):

   - Layer Greek yogurt with fresh berries (blueberries, strawberries, or raspberries) and a sprinkle of chia seeds. This snack provides protein, probiotics, and antioxidants.

   Ingredients:

   - Greek yogurt

   - Fresh berries (blueberries, strawberries, raspberries)

   - Chia seeds

   Instructions:

   1. In a glass or bowl, layer Greek yogurt with fresh berries.

   2. Sprinkle chia seeds on top.

   3. Repeat the layers.

4. Enjoy this protein-packed and antioxidant-rich Greek yogurt parfait.

2. Hummus and Vegetable Sticks (Blood Type B):

- Dip colorful vegetable sticks (carrots, bell peppers, cucumber) into hummus for a satisfying and nutritious snack. Hummus offers plant-based protein and fiber.

Ingredients:

- Hummus

- Carrot sticks

- Bell pepper strips

- Cucumber slices

Instructions:

1. Arrange carrot sticks, bell pepper strips, and cucumber slices on a plate.

2. Dip the vegetables into hummus.

3. Enjoy this crunchy and satisfying hummus and vegetable snack.

3. Mixed Nuts and Dried Fruits (Blood Type O):

   - Create a trail mix with a variety of nuts (almonds, walnuts, or cashews) and dried fruits (apricots, cranberries, or raisins). This snack provides a mix of healthy fats and energy.

   Ingredients:

   - Almonds

   - Walnuts

   - Cashews

   - Dried apricots

   - Cranberries

   - Raisins

   Instructions:

   1. Mix almonds, walnuts, cashews, dried apricots, cranberries, and raisins in a bowl.

   2. Create your trail mix with your preferred ratio of nuts and fruits.

   3. Portion out and enjoy this energy-boosting snack.

4. Rice Cake with Almond Butter (Blood Type AB):

   - Spread almond butter on a brown rice cake for a quick and balanced snack. The combination of healthy fats and whole grains can provide sustained energy.

   Ingredients:

   - Brown rice cake

   - Almond butter

   Instructions:

   1. Spread almond butter on a brown rice cake.

   2. Enjoy this simple and satisfying snack that combines healthy fats with whole grains.

5. Smoothie Bowl with Tropical Fruits (Blood Type B):

   - Blend a smoothie using banana, pineapple, and coconut milk. Pour into a bowl and top with granola, shredded coconut, and a drizzle of honey for a refreshing snack.

   Ingredients:

   - Banana

   - Pineapple chunks

   - Coconut milk

- Granola

- Shredded coconut

- Honey

Instructions:

1. Blend banana, pineapple, and coconut milk until smooth.

2. Pour the smoothie into a bowl.

3. Top with granola, shredded coconut, and a drizzle of honey.

4. Enjoy this refreshing and nutritious smoothie bowl.

Dessert Options:

6. Chia Seed Pudding with Mango (Blood Type A):

- Mix chia seeds with almond milk and let it sit until it thickens. Top with fresh mango cubes for a delicious and nutritious dessert high in omega-3 fatty acids.

Ingredients:

- Chia seeds

- Almond milk

- Mango, diced

Instructions:

1. In a jar, mix chia seeds with almond milk.

2. Refrigerate for a few hours or overnight until it thickens.

3. Layer chia pudding with diced mango.

4. Enjoy this nutrient-rich and naturally sweet chia seed pudding.

7. Dark Chocolate Covered Strawberries (Blood Type O):

- Dip fresh strawberries in dark chocolate for a sweet treat with antioxidants. Dark chocolate in moderation may have potential health benefits.

Ingredients:

- Fresh strawberries

- Dark chocolate (70% cocoa or higher)

Instructions:

1. Melt dark chocolate in a bowl.

2. Dip fresh strawberries into the melted chocolate, coating them partially.

3. Place the chocolate-covered strawberries on a parchment-lined tray.

4. Allow the chocolate to set.

5. Enjoy these antioxidant-rich dark chocolate covered strawberries.

8. Baked Apple with Cinnamon (Blood Type AB):

- Core an apple and sprinkle it with cinnamon. Bake until tender for a warm and comforting dessert that's naturally sweet and rich in fiber.

Ingredients:

- Apples, cored and sliced

- Cinnamon

- Optional: Nutmeg or a drizzle of honey

Instructions:

1. Preheat the oven.

2. Arrange apple slices in a baking dish.

3. Sprinkle with cinnamon and, if desired, nutmeg.

4. Bake until apples are tender.

5. Optional: Drizzle with honey before serving.

9. Coconut Yogurt Parfait with Nuts (Blood Type B):

- Layer coconut yogurt with mixed nuts (such as pistachios and almonds) and a drizzle of honey. This dessert offers a balance of flavors and textures.

Ingredients:

- Coconut yogurt

- Mixed nuts (pistachios, almonds)

- Honey

Instructions:

1. In a glass or bowl, layer coconut yogurt with mixed nuts.

2. Drizzle honey over the top.

3. Repeat the layers.

4. Enjoy this delightful and satisfying coconut yogurt parfait.

10. Avocado Chocolate Mousse (Blood Type O):

- Blend ripe avocado with cocoa powder, a touch of honey, and vanilla extract for a creamy chocolate mousse. This dessert is rich in healthy fats and antioxidants.

Ingredients:

- Ripe avocados

- Cocoa powder

- Honey or maple syrup

- Vanilla extract

Instructions:

1. In a blender, combine ripe avocados, cocoa powder, honey or maple syrup, and vanilla extract.

2. Blend until smooth and creamy.

3. Chill the chocolate avocado mousse in the refrigerator.

4. Serve and savor this rich and healthy chocolate mousse.

Seven day meal plan

Day 1:

- Breakfast: Omelette with Spinach and Turkey

- Lunch: Grilled Chicken Salad with Mixed Greens

- Dinner: Grilled Salmon with Asparagus

Day 2:

- Breakfast: Greek Yogurt Parfait with Berries

- Lunch: Vegetarian Quinoa Bowl

- Dinner: Vegetarian Stir-Fried Tofu and Broccoli

Day 3:

- Breakfast: Smoked Salmon and Avocado Toast

- Lunch: Salmon Sushi Bowl

- Dinner: Turkey and Vegetable Skewers

Day 4:

- Breakfast: Quinoa Breakfast Bowl with Fruit

- Lunch: Chickpea and Vegetable Stir-Fry

- Dinner: Quinoa Stuffed Bell Peppers

Day 5:

- Breakfast: Almond Butter Banana Smoothie

- Lunch: Turkey and Avocado Wrap

- Dinner: Chicken and Vegetable Curry

Day 6:

- Breakfast: Chia Seed Pudding with Coconut Milk

- Lunch: Mediterranean Lentil Salad

- Dinner: Mushroom and Spinach Frittata

Day 7:

- Breakfast: Egg White Veggie Scramble

- Lunch: Shrimp and Veggie Skewers

- Dinner: Vegetarian Broccoli and Tofu Stir-Fry

This is just a sample, so remember that you can adjust these meals according to your preferences.

Conclusion

Dear Readers,

As I reflect on our shared journey through the world of personalized nutrition and the profound impact of the Blood Type Diet, my heart swells with gratitude. It's been a privilege to embark on this adventure alongside you, exploring the intricate dance between our unique blood types and the foods that fuel our bodies.

Your commitment to understanding and embracing the principles of personalized nutrition is nothing short of inspiring. Each step you take toward mindful eating is a testament to your dedication to well-being. Remember, this journey is not about perfection but about progress, and every positive choice you make is a step toward a healthier, more vibrant you.

I want to express my deepest appreciation for your trust and engagement. Your stories, questions, and shared experiences have enriched our collective exploration, creating a community bound by a shared commitment to health and vitality.

As we continue forward, let's carry the lessons learned together and celebrate the beauty of individuality. May your path be illuminated by the choices that honor your unique constitution, bringing you closer to the vitality you deserve.

Wishing you abundant health, joy, and fulfillment on your journey.

With heartfelt gratitude,

Becky Shelby

About the author

Becky Shelby is a passionate advocate for holistic well-being, blending her love for nutrition, health, and lifestyle. With a keen interest in exploring the intersection of dietary choices and individual health, Becky has dedicated herself to researching and understanding how nutrition impacts our bodies, specifically in the context of blood types.

Her journey into the world of nutrition began with a personal quest for optimal health and vitality. Drawing inspiration from her own experiences, Becky has delved into the intricacies of the Blood Type Diet, exploring how tailored nutrition can contribute to overall well-being.

As an author, Becky aims to share her knowledge and insights with a wider audience, simplifying complex nutritional concepts and providing practical guidance for individuals seeking to make informed choices aligned with their blood type. Through her writing, she aspires to empower readers to embark on their own journeys toward a healthier and more balanced lifestyle.

Becky's approach is characterized by a commitment to evidence-based information, an appreciation for diverse dietary needs, and a genuine passion for helping others discover the profound impact of mindful nutrition.

Whether you are new to the concept of blood type-based nutrition or seeking to deepen your understanding, Becky Shelby's work invites you to explore the fascinating and personalized world of the Blood Type Diet.

In addition to her writing, Becky enjoys connecting with her readers through various platforms, sharing tips, recipes, and insights to inspire positive changes in their health and well-being. Her mission is to foster a community of individuals who embrace the transformative power of personalized nutrition on their journey to vibrant health.

My Little Request

If you have gotten to this point, chances are high you
have finished this book.

Thank You for Reading My Book!

I love hearing what you have to say.

I need your input to make the next version of this

book and my future books better.

Please take two minutes now to leave a helpful review
on Amazon letting me know what you thought of the
book

Thanks so much!

- Becky Shelby

www.ingramcontent.com/pod-product-compliance
Lightning Source LLC
Chambersburg PA
CBHW070821280726
48660CB00017B/2329